Fire Alarm Log Book

BUSINESS DETAILS

BUSINESS	
ADDRESS:	
EMAIL:	
PHONE:	

EMERGENCY CONTACT:		CONTACT NUMBER:	

BOOK INFORMATION

CONTINUED FROM BOOK:		CONTINUED TO BOOK:	
BOOK START DATE:		BOOK END DATE:	

NOTES / IMPORTANT INFORMATION

Fire Alarm Log Book

DATE:	SERIAL NUMBER:
LOCATION:	
ALARM CHECKS:	
ACTION REQUIRED:	
INSPECTION TIME:	INSPECTED BY:
COMMENTS:	

DATE:	SERIAL NUMBER:
LOCATION:	
ALARM CHECKS:	
ACTION REQUIRED:	
INSPECTION TIME:	INSPECTED BY:
COMMENTS:	

DATE:	SERIAL NUMBER:
LOCATION:	
ALARM CHECKS:	
ACTION REQUIRED:	
INSPECTION TIME:	INSPECTED BY:
COMMENTS:	

DATE:	SERIAL NUMBER:
LOCATION:	
ALARM CHECKS:	
ACTION REQUIRED:	
INSPECTION TIME:	INSPECTED BY:
COMMENTS:	

Fire Alarm Log Book

DATE:	SERIAL NUMBER:
LOCATION:	
ALARM CHECKS:	
ACTION REQUIRED:	
INSPECTION TIME:	INSPECTED BY:
COMMENTS:	

DATE:	SERIAL NUMBER:
LOCATION:	
ALARM CHECKS:	
ACTION REQUIRED:	
INSPECTION TIME:	INSPECTED BY:
COMMENTS:	

DATE:	SERIAL NUMBER:
LOCATION:	
ALARM CHECKS:	
ACTION REQUIRED:	
INSPECTION TIME:	INSPECTED BY:
COMMENTS:	

DATE:	SERIAL NUMBER:
LOCATION:	
ALARM CHECKS:	
ACTION REQUIRED:	
INSPECTION TIME:	INSPECTED BY:
COMMENTS:	

Fire Alarm Log Book

DATE:	SERIAL NUMBER:
LOCATION:	
ALARM CHECKS:	
ACTION REQUIRED:	
INSPECTION TIME:	INSPECTED BY:
COMMENTS:	

DATE:	SERIAL NUMBER:
LOCATION:	
ALARM CHECKS:	
ACTION REQUIRED:	
INSPECTION TIME:	INSPECTED BY:
COMMENTS:	

DATE:	SERIAL NUMBER:
LOCATION:	
ALARM CHECKS:	
ACTION REQUIRED:	
INSPECTION TIME:	INSPECTED BY:
COMMENTS:	

DATE:	SERIAL NUMBER:
LOCATION:	
ALARM CHECKS:	
ACTION REQUIRED:	
INSPECTION TIME:	INSPECTED BY:
COMMENTS:	

Fire Alarm Log Book

DATE:	SERIAL NUMBER:
LOCATION:	
ALARM CHECKS:	
ACTION REQUIRED:	
INSPECTION TIME:	INSPECTED BY:
COMMENTS:	

DATE:	SERIAL NUMBER:
LOCATION:	
ALARM CHECKS:	
ACTION REQUIRED:	
INSPECTION TIME:	INSPECTED BY:
COMMENTS:	

DATE:	SERIAL NUMBER:
LOCATION:	
ALARM CHECKS:	
ACTION REQUIRED:	
INSPECTION TIME:	INSPECTED BY:
COMMENTS:	

DATE:	SERIAL NUMBER:
LOCATION:	
ALARM CHECKS:	
ACTION REQUIRED:	
INSPECTION TIME:	INSPECTED BY:
COMMENTS:	

Fire Alarm Log Book

DATE:	SERIAL NUMBER:
LOCATION:	
ALARM CHECKS:	
ACTION REQUIRED:	
INSPECTION TIME:	INSPECTED BY:
COMMENTS:	

DATE:	SERIAL NUMBER:
LOCATION:	
ALARM CHECKS:	
ACTION REQUIRED:	
INSPECTION TIME:	INSPECTED BY:
COMMENTS:	

DATE:	SERIAL NUMBER:
LOCATION:	
ALARM CHECKS:	
ACTION REQUIRED:	
INSPECTION TIME:	INSPECTED BY:
COMMENTS:	

DATE:	SERIAL NUMBER:
LOCATION:	
ALARM CHECKS:	
ACTION REQUIRED:	
INSPECTION TIME:	INSPECTED BY:
COMMENTS:	

Fire Alarm Log Book

DATE:	SERIAL NUMBER:
LOCATION:	
ALARM CHECKS:	
ACTION REQUIRED:	
INSPECTION TIME:	INSPECTED BY:
COMMENTS:	

DATE:	SERIAL NUMBER:
LOCATION:	
ALARM CHECKS:	
ACTION REQUIRED:	
INSPECTION TIME:	INSPECTED BY:
COMMENTS:	

DATE:	SERIAL NUMBER:
LOCATION:	
ALARM CHECKS:	
ACTION REQUIRED:	
INSPECTION TIME:	INSPECTED BY:
COMMENTS:	

DATE:	SERIAL NUMBER:
LOCATION:	
ALARM CHECKS:	
ACTION REQUIRED:	
INSPECTION TIME:	INSPECTED BY:
COMMENTS:	

Fire Alarm Log Book

DATE:	SERIAL NUMBER:
LOCATION:	
ALARM CHECKS:	
ACTION REQUIRED:	
INSPECTION TIME:	INSPECTED BY:
COMMENTS:	

DATE:	SERIAL NUMBER:
LOCATION:	
ALARM CHECKS:	
ACTION REQUIRED:	
INSPECTION TIME:	INSPECTED BY:
COMMENTS:	

DATE:	SERIAL NUMBER:
LOCATION:	
ALARM CHECKS:	
ACTION REQUIRED:	
INSPECTION TIME:	INSPECTED BY:
COMMENTS:	

DATE:	SERIAL NUMBER:
LOCATION:	
ALARM CHECKS:	
ACTION REQUIRED:	
INSPECTION TIME:	INSPECTED BY:
COMMENTS:	

Fire Alarm Log Book

DATE:	SERIAL NUMBER:
LOCATION:	
ALARM CHECKS:	
ACTION REQUIRED:	
INSPECTION TIME:	INSPECTED BY:
COMMENTS:	

DATE:	SERIAL NUMBER:
LOCATION:	
ALARM CHECKS:	
ACTION REQUIRED:	
INSPECTION TIME:	INSPECTED BY:
COMMENTS:	

DATE:	SERIAL NUMBER:
LOCATION:	
ALARM CHECKS:	
ACTION REQUIRED:	
INSPECTION TIME:	INSPECTED BY:
COMMENTS:	

DATE:	SERIAL NUMBER:
LOCATION:	
ALARM CHECKS:	
ACTION REQUIRED:	
INSPECTION TIME:	INSPECTED BY:
COMMENTS:	

Fire Alarm Log Book

DATE:	SERIAL NUMBER:
LOCATION:	
ALARM CHECKS:	
ACTION REQUIRED:	
INSPECTION TIME:	INSPECTED BY:
COMMENTS:	

DATE:	SERIAL NUMBER:
LOCATION:	
ALARM CHECKS:	
ACTION REQUIRED:	
INSPECTION TIME:	INSPECTED BY:
COMMENTS:	

DATE:	SERIAL NUMBER:
LOCATION:	
ALARM CHECKS:	
ACTION REQUIRED:	
INSPECTION TIME:	INSPECTED BY:
COMMENTS:	

DATE:	SERIAL NUMBER:
LOCATION:	
ALARM CHECKS:	
ACTION REQUIRED:	
INSPECTION TIME:	INSPECTED BY:
COMMENTS:	

Fire Alarm Log Book

DATE:	SERIAL NUMBER:
LOCATION:	
ALARM CHECKS:	
ACTION REQUIRED:	
INSPECTION TIME:	INSPECTED BY:
COMMENTS:	

DATE:	SERIAL NUMBER:
LOCATION:	
ALARM CHECKS:	
ACTION REQUIRED:	
INSPECTION TIME:	INSPECTED BY:
COMMENTS:	

DATE:	SERIAL NUMBER:
LOCATION:	
ALARM CHECKS:	
ACTION REQUIRED:	
INSPECTION TIME:	INSPECTED BY:
COMMENTS:	

DATE:	SERIAL NUMBER:
LOCATION:	
ALARM CHECKS:	
ACTION REQUIRED:	
INSPECTION TIME:	INSPECTED BY:
COMMENTS:	

Fire Alarm Log Book

DATE:	SERIAL NUMBER:
LOCATION:	
ALARM CHECKS:	
ACTION REQUIRED:	
INSPECTION TIME:	INSPECTED BY:
COMMENTS:	

DATE:	SERIAL NUMBER:
LOCATION:	
ALARM CHECKS:	
ACTION REQUIRED:	
INSPECTION TIME:	INSPECTED BY:
COMMENTS:	

DATE:	SERIAL NUMBER:
LOCATION:	
ALARM CHECKS:	
ACTION REQUIRED:	
INSPECTION TIME:	INSPECTED BY:
COMMENTS:	

DATE:	SERIAL NUMBER:
LOCATION:	
ALARM CHECKS:	
ACTION REQUIRED:	
INSPECTION TIME:	INSPECTED BY:
COMMENTS:	

Fire Alarm Log Book

DATE:	SERIAL NUMBER:
LOCATION:	
ALARM CHECKS:	
ACTION REQUIRED:	
INSPECTION TIME:	INSPECTED BY:
COMMENTS:	

DATE:	SERIAL NUMBER:
LOCATION:	
ALARM CHECKS:	
ACTION REQUIRED:	
INSPECTION TIME:	INSPECTED BY:
COMMENTS:	

DATE:	SERIAL NUMBER:
LOCATION:	
ALARM CHECKS:	
ACTION REQUIRED:	
INSPECTION TIME:	INSPECTED BY:
COMMENTS:	

DATE:	SERIAL NUMBER:
LOCATION:	
ALARM CHECKS:	
ACTION REQUIRED:	
INSPECTION TIME:	INSPECTED BY:
COMMENTS:	

Fire Alarm Log Book

DATE:	SERIAL NUMBER:
LOCATION:	
ALARM CHECKS:	
ACTION REQUIRED:	
INSPECTION TIME:	INSPECTED BY:
COMMENTS:	

DATE:	SERIAL NUMBER:
LOCATION:	
ALARM CHECKS:	
ACTION REQUIRED:	
INSPECTION TIME:	INSPECTED BY:
COMMENTS:	

DATE:	SERIAL NUMBER:
LOCATION:	
ALARM CHECKS:	
ACTION REQUIRED:	
INSPECTION TIME:	INSPECTED BY:
COMMENTS:	

DATE:	SERIAL NUMBER:
LOCATION:	
ALARM CHECKS:	
ACTION REQUIRED:	
INSPECTION TIME:	INSPECTED BY:
COMMENTS:	

Fire Alarm Log Book

DATE:	SERIAL NUMBER:
LOCATION:	
ALARM CHECKS:	
ACTION REQUIRED:	
INSPECTION TIME:	INSPECTED BY:
COMMENTS:	

DATE:	SERIAL NUMBER:
LOCATION:	
ALARM CHECKS:	
ACTION REQUIRED:	
INSPECTION TIME:	INSPECTED BY:
COMMENTS:	

DATE:	SERIAL NUMBER:
LOCATION:	
ALARM CHECKS:	
ACTION REQUIRED:	
INSPECTION TIME:	INSPECTED BY:
COMMENTS:	

DATE:	SERIAL NUMBER:
LOCATION:	
ALARM CHECKS:	
ACTION REQUIRED:	
INSPECTION TIME:	INSPECTED BY:
COMMENTS:	

Fire Alarm Log Book

DATE:	SERIAL NUMBER:
LOCATION:	
ALARM CHECKS:	
ACTION REQUIRED:	
INSPECTION TIME:	INSPECTED BY:
COMMENTS:	

DATE:	SERIAL NUMBER:
LOCATION:	
ALARM CHECKS:	
ACTION REQUIRED:	
INSPECTION TIME:	INSPECTED BY:
COMMENTS:	

DATE:	SERIAL NUMBER:
LOCATION:	
ALARM CHECKS:	
ACTION REQUIRED:	
INSPECTION TIME:	INSPECTED BY:
COMMENTS:	

DATE:	SERIAL NUMBER:
LOCATION:	
ALARM CHECKS:	
ACTION REQUIRED:	
INSPECTION TIME:	INSPECTED BY:
COMMENTS:	

Fire Alarm Log Book

DATE:	SERIAL NUMBER:
LOCATION:	
ALARM CHECKS:	
ACTION REQUIRED:	
INSPECTION TIME:	INSPECTED BY:
COMMENTS:	

DATE:	SERIAL NUMBER:
LOCATION:	
ALARM CHECKS:	
ACTION REQUIRED:	
INSPECTION TIME:	INSPECTED BY:
COMMENTS:	

DATE:	SERIAL NUMBER:
LOCATION:	
ALARM CHECKS:	
ACTION REQUIRED:	
INSPECTION TIME:	INSPECTED BY:
COMMENTS:	

DATE:	SERIAL NUMBER:
LOCATION:	
ALARM CHECKS:	
ACTION REQUIRED:	
INSPECTION TIME:	INSPECTED BY:
COMMENTS:	

Fire Alarm Log Book

DATE:	SERIAL NUMBER:
LOCATION:	
ALARM CHECKS:	
ACTION REQUIRED:	
INSPECTION TIME:	INSPECTED BY:
COMMENTS:	

DATE:	SERIAL NUMBER:
LOCATION:	
ALARM CHECKS:	
ACTION REQUIRED:	
INSPECTION TIME:	INSPECTED BY:
COMMENTS:	

DATE:	SERIAL NUMBER:
LOCATION:	
ALARM CHECKS:	
ACTION REQUIRED:	
INSPECTION TIME:	INSPECTED BY:
COMMENTS:	

DATE:	SERIAL NUMBER:
LOCATION:	
ALARM CHECKS:	
ACTION REQUIRED:	
INSPECTION TIME:	INSPECTED BY:
COMMENTS:	

Fire Alarm Log Book

DATE:	SERIAL NUMBER:
LOCATION:	
ALARM CHECKS:	
ACTION REQUIRED:	
INSPECTION TIME:	INSPECTED BY:
COMMENTS:	

DATE:	SERIAL NUMBER:
LOCATION:	
ALARM CHECKS:	
ACTION REQUIRED:	
INSPECTION TIME:	INSPECTED BY:
COMMENTS:	

DATE:	SERIAL NUMBER:
LOCATION:	
ALARM CHECKS:	
ACTION REQUIRED:	
INSPECTION TIME:	INSPECTED BY:
COMMENTS:	

DATE:	SERIAL NUMBER:
LOCATION:	
ALARM CHECKS:	
ACTION REQUIRED:	
INSPECTION TIME:	INSPECTED BY:
COMMENTS:	

Fire Alarm Log Book

DATE:	SERIAL NUMBER:
LOCATION:	
ALARM CHECKS:	
ACTION REQUIRED:	
INSPECTION TIME:	INSPECTED BY:
COMMENTS:	

DATE:	SERIAL NUMBER:
LOCATION:	
ALARM CHECKS:	
ACTION REQUIRED:	
INSPECTION TIME:	INSPECTED BY:
COMMENTS:	

DATE:	SERIAL NUMBER:
LOCATION:	
ALARM CHECKS:	
ACTION REQUIRED:	
INSPECTION TIME:	INSPECTED BY:
COMMENTS:	

DATE:	SERIAL NUMBER:
LOCATION:	
ALARM CHECKS:	
ACTION REQUIRED:	
INSPECTION TIME:	INSPECTED BY:
COMMENTS:	

Fire Alarm Log Book

DATE:	SERIAL NUMBER:
LOCATION:	
ALARM CHECKS:	
ACTION REQUIRED:	
INSPECTION TIME:	INSPECTED BY:
COMMENTS:	

DATE:	SERIAL NUMBER:
LOCATION:	
ALARM CHECKS:	
ACTION REQUIRED:	
INSPECTION TIME:	INSPECTED BY:
COMMENTS:	

DATE:	SERIAL NUMBER:
LOCATION:	
ALARM CHECKS:	
ACTION REQUIRED:	
INSPECTION TIME:	INSPECTED BY:
COMMENTS:	

DATE:	SERIAL NUMBER:
LOCATION:	
ALARM CHECKS:	
ACTION REQUIRED:	
INSPECTION TIME:	INSPECTED BY:
COMMENTS:	

Fire Alarm Log Book

DATE:	SERIAL NUMBER:
LOCATION:	
ALARM CHECKS:	
ACTION REQUIRED:	
INSPECTION TIME:	INSPECTED BY:
COMMENTS:	

DATE:	SERIAL NUMBER:
LOCATION:	
ALARM CHECKS:	
ACTION REQUIRED:	
INSPECTION TIME:	INSPECTED BY:
COMMENTS:	

DATE:	SERIAL NUMBER:
LOCATION:	
ALARM CHECKS:	
ACTION REQUIRED:	
INSPECTION TIME:	INSPECTED BY:
COMMENTS:	

DATE:	SERIAL NUMBER:
LOCATION:	
ALARM CHECKS:	
ACTION REQUIRED:	
INSPECTION TIME:	INSPECTED BY:
COMMENTS:	

Fire Alarm Log Book

DATE:	SERIAL NUMBER:
LOCATION:	
ALARM CHECKS:	
ACTION REQUIRED:	
INSPECTION TIME:	INSPECTED BY:
COMMENTS:	

DATE:	SERIAL NUMBER:
LOCATION:	
ALARM CHECKS:	
ACTION REQUIRED:	
INSPECTION TIME:	INSPECTED BY:
COMMENTS:	

DATE:	SERIAL NUMBER:
LOCATION:	
ALARM CHECKS:	
ACTION REQUIRED:	
INSPECTION TIME:	INSPECTED BY:
COMMENTS:	

DATE:	SERIAL NUMBER:
LOCATION:	
ALARM CHECKS:	
ACTION REQUIRED:	
INSPECTION TIME:	INSPECTED BY:
COMMENTS:	

Fire Alarm Log Book

DATE:	SERIAL NUMBER:
LOCATION:	
ALARM CHECKS:	
ACTION REQUIRED:	
INSPECTION TIME:	INSPECTED BY:
COMMENTS:	

DATE:	SERIAL NUMBER:
LOCATION:	
ALARM CHECKS:	
ACTION REQUIRED:	
INSPECTION TIME:	INSPECTED BY:
COMMENTS:	

DATE:	SERIAL NUMBER:
LOCATION:	
ALARM CHECKS:	
ACTION REQUIRED:	
INSPECTION TIME:	INSPECTED BY:
COMMENTS:	

DATE:	SERIAL NUMBER:
LOCATION:	
ALARM CHECKS:	
ACTION REQUIRED:	
INSPECTION TIME:	INSPECTED BY:
COMMENTS:	

Fire Alarm Log Book

DATE:	SERIAL NUMBER:
LOCATION:	
ALARM CHECKS:	
ACTION REQUIRED:	
INSPECTION TIME:	INSPECTED BY:
COMMENTS:	

DATE:	SERIAL NUMBER:
LOCATION:	
ALARM CHECKS:	
ACTION REQUIRED:	
INSPECTION TIME:	INSPECTED BY:
COMMENTS:	

DATE:	SERIAL NUMBER:
LOCATION:	
ALARM CHECKS:	
ACTION REQUIRED:	
INSPECTION TIME:	INSPECTED BY:
COMMENTS:	

DATE:	SERIAL NUMBER:
LOCATION:	
ALARM CHECKS:	
ACTION REQUIRED:	
INSPECTION TIME:	INSPECTED BY:
COMMENTS:	

Fire Alarm Log Book

DATE:	SERIAL NUMBER:
LOCATION:	
ALARM CHECKS:	
ACTION REQUIRED:	
INSPECTION TIME:	INSPECTED BY:
COMMENTS:	

DATE:	SERIAL NUMBER:
LOCATION:	
ALARM CHECKS:	
ACTION REQUIRED:	
INSPECTION TIME:	INSPECTED BY:
COMMENTS:	

DATE:	SERIAL NUMBER:
LOCATION:	
ALARM CHECKS:	
ACTION REQUIRED:	
INSPECTION TIME:	INSPECTED BY:
COMMENTS:	

DATE:	SERIAL NUMBER:
LOCATION:	
ALARM CHECKS:	
ACTION REQUIRED:	
INSPECTION TIME:	INSPECTED BY:
COMMENTS:	

Fire Alarm Log Book

DATE:	SERIAL NUMBER:
LOCATION:	
ALARM CHECKS:	
ACTION REQUIRED:	
INSPECTION TIME:	INSPECTED BY:
COMMENTS:	

DATE:	SERIAL NUMBER:
LOCATION:	
ALARM CHECKS:	
ACTION REQUIRED:	
INSPECTION TIME:	INSPECTED BY:
COMMENTS:	

DATE:	SERIAL NUMBER:
LOCATION:	
ALARM CHECKS:	
ACTION REQUIRED:	
INSPECTION TIME:	INSPECTED BY:
COMMENTS:	

DATE:	SERIAL NUMBER:
LOCATION:	
ALARM CHECKS:	
ACTION REQUIRED:	
INSPECTION TIME:	INSPECTED BY:
COMMENTS:	

Fire Alarm Log Book

DATE:	SERIAL NUMBER:
LOCATION:	
ALARM CHECKS:	
ACTION REQUIRED:	
INSPECTION TIME:	INSPECTED BY:
COMMENTS:	

DATE:	SERIAL NUMBER:
LOCATION:	
ALARM CHECKS:	
ACTION REQUIRED:	
INSPECTION TIME:	INSPECTED BY:
COMMENTS:	

DATE:	SERIAL NUMBER:
LOCATION:	
ALARM CHECKS:	
ACTION REQUIRED:	
INSPECTION TIME:	INSPECTED BY:
COMMENTS:	

DATE:	SERIAL NUMBER:
LOCATION:	
ALARM CHECKS:	
ACTION REQUIRED:	
INSPECTION TIME:	INSPECTED BY:
COMMENTS:	

Fire Alarm Log Book

DATE:	SERIAL NUMBER:
LOCATION:	
ALARM CHECKS:	
ACTION REQUIRED:	
INSPECTION TIME:	INSPECTED BY:
COMMENTS:	

DATE:	SERIAL NUMBER:
LOCATION:	
ALARM CHECKS:	
ACTION REQUIRED:	
INSPECTION TIME:	INSPECTED BY:
COMMENTS:	

DATE:	SERIAL NUMBER:
LOCATION:	
ALARM CHECKS:	
ACTION REQUIRED:	
INSPECTION TIME:	INSPECTED BY:
COMMENTS:	

DATE:	SERIAL NUMBER:
LOCATION:	
ALARM CHECKS:	
ACTION REQUIRED:	
INSPECTION TIME:	INSPECTED BY:
COMMENTS:	

Fire Alarm Log Book

DATE:	SERIAL NUMBER:
LOCATION:	
ALARM CHECKS:	
ACTION REQUIRED:	
INSPECTION TIME:	INSPECTED BY:
COMMENTS:	

DATE:	SERIAL NUMBER:
LOCATION:	
ALARM CHECKS:	
ACTION REQUIRED:	
INSPECTION TIME:	INSPECTED BY:
COMMENTS:	

DATE:	SERIAL NUMBER:
LOCATION:	
ALARM CHECKS:	
ACTION REQUIRED:	
INSPECTION TIME:	INSPECTED BY:
COMMENTS:	

DATE:	SERIAL NUMBER:
LOCATION:	
ALARM CHECKS:	
ACTION REQUIRED:	
INSPECTION TIME:	INSPECTED BY:
COMMENTS:	

Fire Alarm Log Book

DATE:	SERIAL NUMBER:
LOCATION:	
ALARM CHECKS:	
ACTION REQUIRED:	
INSPECTION TIME:	INSPECTED BY:
COMMENTS:	

DATE:	SERIAL NUMBER:
LOCATION:	
ALARM CHECKS:	
ACTION REQUIRED:	
INSPECTION TIME:	INSPECTED BY:
COMMENTS:	

DATE:	SERIAL NUMBER:
LOCATION:	
ALARM CHECKS:	
ACTION REQUIRED:	
INSPECTION TIME:	INSPECTED BY:
COMMENTS:	

DATE:	SERIAL NUMBER:
LOCATION:	
ALARM CHECKS:	
ACTION REQUIRED:	
INSPECTION TIME:	INSPECTED BY:
COMMENTS:	

Fire Alarm Log Book

DATE:	SERIAL NUMBER:
LOCATION:	
ALARM CHECKS:	
ACTION REQUIRED:	
INSPECTION TIME:	INSPECTED BY:
COMMENTS:	

DATE:	SERIAL NUMBER:
LOCATION:	
ALARM CHECKS:	
ACTION REQUIRED:	
INSPECTION TIME:	INSPECTED BY:
COMMENTS:	

DATE:	SERIAL NUMBER:
LOCATION:	
ALARM CHECKS:	
ACTION REQUIRED:	
INSPECTION TIME:	INSPECTED BY:
COMMENTS:	

DATE:	SERIAL NUMBER:
LOCATION:	
ALARM CHECKS:	
ACTION REQUIRED:	
INSPECTION TIME:	INSPECTED BY:
COMMENTS:	

Fire Alarm Log Book

DATE:	SERIAL NUMBER:
LOCATION:	
ALARM CHECKS:	
ACTION REQUIRED:	
INSPECTION TIME:	INSPECTED BY:
COMMENTS:	

DATE:	SERIAL NUMBER:
LOCATION:	
ALARM CHECKS:	
ACTION REQUIRED:	
INSPECTION TIME:	INSPECTED BY:
COMMENTS:	

DATE:	SERIAL NUMBER:
LOCATION:	
ALARM CHECKS:	
ACTION REQUIRED:	
INSPECTION TIME:	INSPECTED BY:
COMMENTS:	

DATE:	SERIAL NUMBER:
LOCATION:	
ALARM CHECKS:	
ACTION REQUIRED:	
INSPECTION TIME:	INSPECTED BY:
COMMENTS:	

Fire Alarm Log Book

DATE:	SERIAL NUMBER:
LOCATION:	
ALARM CHECKS:	
ACTION REQUIRED:	
INSPECTION TIME:	INSPECTED BY:
COMMENTS:	

DATE:	SERIAL NUMBER:
LOCATION:	
ALARM CHECKS:	
ACTION REQUIRED:	
INSPECTION TIME:	INSPECTED BY:
COMMENTS:	

DATE:	SERIAL NUMBER:
LOCATION:	
ALARM CHECKS:	
ACTION REQUIRED:	
INSPECTION TIME:	INSPECTED BY:
COMMENTS:	

DATE:	SERIAL NUMBER:
LOCATION:	
ALARM CHECKS:	
ACTION REQUIRED:	
INSPECTION TIME:	INSPECTED BY:
COMMENTS:	

Fire Alarm Log Book

DATE:	SERIAL NUMBER:
LOCATION:	
ALARM CHECKS:	
ACTION REQUIRED:	
INSPECTION TIME:	INSPECTED BY:
COMMENTS:	

DATE:	SERIAL NUMBER:
LOCATION:	
ALARM CHECKS:	
ACTION REQUIRED:	
INSPECTION TIME:	INSPECTED BY:
COMMENTS:	

DATE:	SERIAL NUMBER:
LOCATION:	
ALARM CHECKS:	
ACTION REQUIRED:	
INSPECTION TIME:	INSPECTED BY:
COMMENTS:	

DATE:	SERIAL NUMBER:
LOCATION:	
ALARM CHECKS:	
ACTION REQUIRED:	
INSPECTION TIME:	INSPECTED BY:
COMMENTS:	

Fire Alarm Log Book

DATE:	SERIAL NUMBER:
LOCATION:	
ALARM CHECKS:	
ACTION REQUIRED:	
INSPECTION TIME:	INSPECTED BY:
COMMENTS:	

DATE:	SERIAL NUMBER:
LOCATION:	
ALARM CHECKS:	
ACTION REQUIRED:	
INSPECTION TIME:	INSPECTED BY:
COMMENTS:	

DATE:	SERIAL NUMBER:
LOCATION:	
ALARM CHECKS:	
ACTION REQUIRED:	
INSPECTION TIME:	INSPECTED BY:
COMMENTS:	

DATE:	SERIAL NUMBER:
LOCATION:	
ALARM CHECKS:	
ACTION REQUIRED:	
INSPECTION TIME:	INSPECTED BY:
COMMENTS:	

Fire Alarm Log Book

DATE:	SERIAL NUMBER:
LOCATION:	
ALARM CHECKS:	
ACTION REQUIRED:	
INSPECTION TIME:	INSPECTED BY:
COMMENTS:	

DATE:	SERIAL NUMBER:
LOCATION:	
ALARM CHECKS:	
ACTION REQUIRED:	
INSPECTION TIME:	INSPECTED BY:
COMMENTS:	

DATE:	SERIAL NUMBER:
LOCATION:	
ALARM CHECKS:	
ACTION REQUIRED:	
INSPECTION TIME:	INSPECTED BY:
COMMENTS:	

DATE:	SERIAL NUMBER:
LOCATION:	
ALARM CHECKS:	
ACTION REQUIRED:	
INSPECTION TIME:	INSPECTED BY:
COMMENTS:	

Fire Alarm Log Book

DATE:	SERIAL NUMBER:
LOCATION:	
ALARM CHECKS:	
ACTION REQUIRED:	
INSPECTION TIME:	INSPECTED BY:
COMMENTS:	

DATE:	SERIAL NUMBER:
LOCATION:	
ALARM CHECKS:	
ACTION REQUIRED:	
INSPECTION TIME:	INSPECTED BY:
COMMENTS:	

DATE:	SERIAL NUMBER:
LOCATION:	
ALARM CHECKS:	
ACTION REQUIRED:	
INSPECTION TIME:	INSPECTED BY:
COMMENTS:	

DATE:	SERIAL NUMBER:
LOCATION:	
ALARM CHECKS:	
ACTION REQUIRED:	
INSPECTION TIME:	INSPECTED BY:
COMMENTS:	

Fire Alarm Log Book

DATE:	SERIAL NUMBER:
LOCATION:	
ALARM CHECKS:	
ACTION REQUIRED:	
INSPECTION TIME:	INSPECTED BY:
COMMENTS:	

DATE:	SERIAL NUMBER:
LOCATION:	
ALARM CHECKS:	
ACTION REQUIRED:	
INSPECTION TIME:	INSPECTED BY:
COMMENTS:	

DATE:	SERIAL NUMBER:
LOCATION:	
ALARM CHECKS:	
ACTION REQUIRED:	
INSPECTION TIME:	INSPECTED BY:
COMMENTS:	

DATE:	SERIAL NUMBER:
LOCATION:	
ALARM CHECKS:	
ACTION REQUIRED:	
INSPECTION TIME:	INSPECTED BY:
COMMENTS:	

Fire Alarm Log Book

DATE:	SERIAL NUMBER:
LOCATION:	
ALARM CHECKS:	
ACTION REQUIRED:	
INSPECTION TIME:	INSPECTED BY:
COMMENTS:	

DATE:	SERIAL NUMBER:
LOCATION:	
ALARM CHECKS:	
ACTION REQUIRED:	
INSPECTION TIME:	INSPECTED BY:
COMMENTS:	

DATE:	SERIAL NUMBER:
LOCATION:	
ALARM CHECKS:	
ACTION REQUIRED:	
INSPECTION TIME:	INSPECTED BY:
COMMENTS:	

DATE:	SERIAL NUMBER:
LOCATION:	
ALARM CHECKS:	
ACTION REQUIRED:	
INSPECTION TIME:	INSPECTED BY:
COMMENTS:	

Fire Alarm Log Book

DATE:	SERIAL NUMBER:
LOCATION:	
ALARM CHECKS:	
ACTION REQUIRED:	
INSPECTION TIME:	INSPECTED BY:
COMMENTS:	

DATE:	SERIAL NUMBER:
LOCATION:	
ALARM CHECKS:	
ACTION REQUIRED:	
INSPECTION TIME:	INSPECTED BY:
COMMENTS:	

DATE:	SERIAL NUMBER:
LOCATION:	
ALARM CHECKS:	
ACTION REQUIRED:	
INSPECTION TIME:	INSPECTED BY:
COMMENTS:	

DATE:	SERIAL NUMBER:
LOCATION:	
ALARM CHECKS:	
ACTION REQUIRED:	
INSPECTION TIME:	INSPECTED BY:
COMMENTS:	

Fire Alarm Log Book

DATE:	SERIAL NUMBER:
LOCATION:	
ALARM CHECKS:	
ACTION REQUIRED:	
INSPECTION TIME:	INSPECTED BY:
COMMENTS:	

DATE:	SERIAL NUMBER:
LOCATION:	
ALARM CHECKS:	
ACTION REQUIRED:	
INSPECTION TIME:	INSPECTED BY:
COMMENTS:	

DATE:	SERIAL NUMBER:
LOCATION:	
ALARM CHECKS:	
ACTION REQUIRED:	
INSPECTION TIME:	INSPECTED BY:
COMMENTS:	

DATE:	SERIAL NUMBER:
LOCATION:	
ALARM CHECKS:	
ACTION REQUIRED:	
INSPECTION TIME:	INSPECTED BY:
COMMENTS:	

Fire Alarm Log Book

DATE:	SERIAL NUMBER:
LOCATION:	
ALARM CHECKS:	
ACTION REQUIRED:	
INSPECTION TIME:	INSPECTED BY:
COMMENTS:	

DATE:	SERIAL NUMBER:
LOCATION:	
ALARM CHECKS:	
ACTION REQUIRED:	
INSPECTION TIME:	INSPECTED BY:
COMMENTS:	

DATE:	SERIAL NUMBER:
LOCATION:	
ALARM CHECKS:	
ACTION REQUIRED:	
INSPECTION TIME:	INSPECTED BY:
COMMENTS:	

DATE:	SERIAL NUMBER:
LOCATION:	
ALARM CHECKS:	
ACTION REQUIRED:	
INSPECTION TIME:	INSPECTED BY:
COMMENTS:	

Fire Alarm Log Book

DATE:	SERIAL NUMBER:
LOCATION:	
ALARM CHECKS:	
ACTION REQUIRED:	
INSPECTION TIME:	INSPECTED BY:
COMMENTS:	

DATE:	SERIAL NUMBER:
LOCATION:	
ALARM CHECKS:	
ACTION REQUIRED:	
INSPECTION TIME:	INSPECTED BY:
COMMENTS:	

DATE:	SERIAL NUMBER:
LOCATION:	
ALARM CHECKS:	
ACTION REQUIRED:	
INSPECTION TIME:	INSPECTED BY:
COMMENTS:	

DATE:	SERIAL NUMBER:
LOCATION:	
ALARM CHECKS:	
ACTION REQUIRED:	
INSPECTION TIME:	INSPECTED BY:
COMMENTS:	

Fire Alarm Log Book

DATE:	SERIAL NUMBER:
LOCATION:	
ALARM CHECKS:	
ACTION REQUIRED:	
INSPECTION TIME:	INSPECTED BY:
COMMENTS:	

DATE:	SERIAL NUMBER:
LOCATION:	
ALARM CHECKS:	
ACTION REQUIRED:	
INSPECTION TIME:	INSPECTED BY:
COMMENTS:	

DATE:	SERIAL NUMBER:
LOCATION:	
ALARM CHECKS:	
ACTION REQUIRED:	
INSPECTION TIME:	INSPECTED BY:
COMMENTS:	

DATE:	SERIAL NUMBER:
LOCATION:	
ALARM CHECKS:	
ACTION REQUIRED:	
INSPECTION TIME:	INSPECTED BY:
COMMENTS:	

Fire Alarm Log Book

DATE:	SERIAL NUMBER:
LOCATION:	
ALARM CHECKS:	
ACTION REQUIRED:	
INSPECTION TIME:	INSPECTED BY:
COMMENTS:	

DATE:	SERIAL NUMBER:
LOCATION:	
ALARM CHECKS:	
ACTION REQUIRED:	
INSPECTION TIME:	INSPECTED BY:
COMMENTS:	

DATE:	SERIAL NUMBER:
LOCATION:	
ALARM CHECKS:	
ACTION REQUIRED:	
INSPECTION TIME:	INSPECTED BY:
COMMENTS:	

DATE:	SERIAL NUMBER:
LOCATION:	
ALARM CHECKS:	
ACTION REQUIRED:	
INSPECTION TIME:	INSPECTED BY:
COMMENTS:	

Fire Alarm Log Book

DATE:	SERIAL NUMBER:
LOCATION:	
ALARM CHECKS:	
ACTION REQUIRED:	
INSPECTION TIME:	INSPECTED BY:
COMMENTS:	

DATE:	SERIAL NUMBER:
LOCATION:	
ALARM CHECKS:	
ACTION REQUIRED:	
INSPECTION TIME:	INSPECTED BY:
COMMENTS:	

DATE:	SERIAL NUMBER:
LOCATION:	
ALARM CHECKS:	
ACTION REQUIRED:	
INSPECTION TIME:	INSPECTED BY:
COMMENTS:	

DATE:	SERIAL NUMBER:
LOCATION:	
ALARM CHECKS:	
ACTION REQUIRED:	
INSPECTION TIME:	INSPECTED BY:
COMMENTS:	

Fire Alarm Log Book

DATE:	SERIAL NUMBER:
LOCATION:	
ALARM CHECKS:	
ACTION REQUIRED:	
INSPECTION TIME:	INSPECTED BY:
COMMENTS:	

DATE:	SERIAL NUMBER:
LOCATION:	
ALARM CHECKS:	
ACTION REQUIRED:	
INSPECTION TIME:	INSPECTED BY:
COMMENTS:	

DATE:	SERIAL NUMBER:
LOCATION:	
ALARM CHECKS:	
ACTION REQUIRED:	
INSPECTION TIME:	INSPECTED BY:
COMMENTS:	

DATE:	SERIAL NUMBER:
LOCATION:	
ALARM CHECKS:	
ACTION REQUIRED:	
INSPECTION TIME:	INSPECTED BY:
COMMENTS:	

Fire Alarm Log Book

DATE:	SERIAL NUMBER:
LOCATION:	
ALARM CHECKS:	
ACTION REQUIRED:	
INSPECTION TIME:	INSPECTED BY:
COMMENTS:	

DATE:	SERIAL NUMBER:
LOCATION:	
ALARM CHECKS:	
ACTION REQUIRED:	
INSPECTION TIME:	INSPECTED BY:
COMMENTS:	

DATE:	SERIAL NUMBER:
LOCATION:	
ALARM CHECKS:	
ACTION REQUIRED:	
INSPECTION TIME:	INSPECTED BY:
COMMENTS:	

DATE:	SERIAL NUMBER:
LOCATION:	
ALARM CHECKS:	
ACTION REQUIRED:	
INSPECTION TIME:	INSPECTED BY:
COMMENTS:	

Fire Alarm Log Book

DATE:	SERIAL NUMBER:
LOCATION:	
ALARM CHECKS:	
ACTION REQUIRED:	
INSPECTION TIME:	INSPECTED BY:
COMMENTS:	

DATE:	SERIAL NUMBER:
LOCATION:	
ALARM CHECKS:	
ACTION REQUIRED:	
INSPECTION TIME:	INSPECTED BY:
COMMENTS:	

DATE:	SERIAL NUMBER:
LOCATION:	
ALARM CHECKS:	
ACTION REQUIRED:	
INSPECTION TIME:	INSPECTED BY:
COMMENTS:	

DATE:	SERIAL NUMBER:
LOCATION:	
ALARM CHECKS:	
ACTION REQUIRED:	
INSPECTION TIME:	INSPECTED BY:
COMMENTS:	

Fire Alarm Log Book

DATE:	SERIAL NUMBER:
LOCATION:	
ALARM CHECKS:	
ACTION REQUIRED:	
INSPECTION TIME:	INSPECTED BY:
COMMENTS:	

DATE:	SERIAL NUMBER:
LOCATION:	
ALARM CHECKS:	
ACTION REQUIRED:	
INSPECTION TIME:	INSPECTED BY:
COMMENTS:	

DATE:	SERIAL NUMBER:
LOCATION:	
ALARM CHECKS:	
ACTION REQUIRED:	
INSPECTION TIME:	INSPECTED BY:
COMMENTS:	

DATE:	SERIAL NUMBER:
LOCATION:	
ALARM CHECKS:	
ACTION REQUIRED:	
INSPECTION TIME:	INSPECTED BY:
COMMENTS:	

Fire Alarm Log Book

DATE:	SERIAL NUMBER:
LOCATION:	
ALARM CHECKS:	
ACTION REQUIRED:	
INSPECTION TIME:	INSPECTED BY:
COMMENTS:	

DATE:	SERIAL NUMBER:
LOCATION:	
ALARM CHECKS:	
ACTION REQUIRED:	
INSPECTION TIME:	INSPECTED BY:
COMMENTS:	

DATE:	SERIAL NUMBER:
LOCATION:	
ALARM CHECKS:	
ACTION REQUIRED:	
INSPECTION TIME:	INSPECTED BY:
COMMENTS:	

DATE:	SERIAL NUMBER:
LOCATION:	
ALARM CHECKS:	
ACTION REQUIRED:	
INSPECTION TIME:	INSPECTED BY:
COMMENTS:	

Fire Alarm Log Book

DATE:	SERIAL NUMBER:
LOCATION:	
ALARM CHECKS:	
ACTION REQUIRED:	
INSPECTION TIME:	INSPECTED BY:
COMMENTS:	

DATE:	SERIAL NUMBER:
LOCATION:	
ALARM CHECKS:	
ACTION REQUIRED:	
INSPECTION TIME:	INSPECTED BY:
COMMENTS:	

DATE:	SERIAL NUMBER:
LOCATION:	
ALARM CHECKS:	
ACTION REQUIRED:	
INSPECTION TIME:	INSPECTED BY:
COMMENTS:	

DATE:	SERIAL NUMBER:
LOCATION:	
ALARM CHECKS:	
ACTION REQUIRED:	
INSPECTION TIME:	INSPECTED BY:
COMMENTS:	

Fire Alarm Log Book

DATE:	SERIAL NUMBER:
LOCATION:	
ALARM CHECKS:	
ACTION REQUIRED:	
INSPECTION TIME:	INSPECTED BY:
COMMENTS:	

DATE:	SERIAL NUMBER:
LOCATION:	
ALARM CHECKS:	
ACTION REQUIRED:	
INSPECTION TIME:	INSPECTED BY:
COMMENTS:	

DATE:	SERIAL NUMBER:
LOCATION:	
ALARM CHECKS:	
ACTION REQUIRED:	
INSPECTION TIME:	INSPECTED BY:
COMMENTS:	

DATE:	SERIAL NUMBER:
LOCATION:	
ALARM CHECKS:	
ACTION REQUIRED:	
INSPECTION TIME:	INSPECTED BY:
COMMENTS:	

Fire Alarm Log Book

DATE:	SERIAL NUMBER:
LOCATION:	
ALARM CHECKS:	
ACTION REQUIRED:	
INSPECTION TIME:	INSPECTED BY:
COMMENTS:	

DATE:	SERIAL NUMBER:
LOCATION:	
ALARM CHECKS:	
ACTION REQUIRED:	
INSPECTION TIME:	INSPECTED BY:
COMMENTS:	

DATE:	SERIAL NUMBER:
LOCATION:	
ALARM CHECKS:	
ACTION REQUIRED:	
INSPECTION TIME:	INSPECTED BY:
COMMENTS:	

DATE:	SERIAL NUMBER:
LOCATION:	
ALARM CHECKS:	
ACTION REQUIRED:	
INSPECTION TIME:	INSPECTED BY:
COMMENTS:	

Fire Alarm Log Book

DATE:	SERIAL NUMBER:
LOCATION:	
ALARM CHECKS:	
ACTION REQUIRED:	
INSPECTION TIME:	INSPECTED BY:
COMMENTS:	

DATE:	SERIAL NUMBER:
LOCATION:	
ALARM CHECKS:	
ACTION REQUIRED:	
INSPECTION TIME:	INSPECTED BY:
COMMENTS:	

DATE:	SERIAL NUMBER:
LOCATION:	
ALARM CHECKS:	
ACTION REQUIRED:	
INSPECTION TIME:	INSPECTED BY:
COMMENTS:	

DATE:	SERIAL NUMBER:
LOCATION:	
ALARM CHECKS:	
ACTION REQUIRED:	
INSPECTION TIME:	INSPECTED BY:
COMMENTS:	

Fire Alarm Log Book

DATE:	SERIAL NUMBER:
LOCATION:	
ALARM CHECKS:	
ACTION REQUIRED:	
INSPECTION TIME:	INSPECTED BY:
COMMENTS:	

DATE:	SERIAL NUMBER:
LOCATION:	
ALARM CHECKS:	
ACTION REQUIRED:	
INSPECTION TIME:	INSPECTED BY:
COMMENTS:	

DATE:	SERIAL NUMBER:
LOCATION:	
ALARM CHECKS:	
ACTION REQUIRED:	
INSPECTION TIME:	INSPECTED BY:
COMMENTS:	

DATE:	SERIAL NUMBER:
LOCATION:	
ALARM CHECKS:	
ACTION REQUIRED:	
INSPECTION TIME:	INSPECTED BY:
COMMENTS:	

Fire Alarm Log Book

DATE:	SERIAL NUMBER:
LOCATION:	
ALARM CHECKS:	
ACTION REQUIRED:	
INSPECTION TIME:	INSPECTED BY:
COMMENTS:	

DATE:	SERIAL NUMBER:
LOCATION:	
ALARM CHECKS:	
ACTION REQUIRED:	
INSPECTION TIME:	INSPECTED BY:
COMMENTS:	

DATE:	SERIAL NUMBER:
LOCATION:	
ALARM CHECKS:	
ACTION REQUIRED:	
INSPECTION TIME:	INSPECTED BY:
COMMENTS:	

DATE:	SERIAL NUMBER:
LOCATION:	
ALARM CHECKS:	
ACTION REQUIRED:	
INSPECTION TIME:	INSPECTED BY:
COMMENTS:	

Fire Alarm Log Book

DATE:	SERIAL NUMBER:
LOCATION:	
ALARM CHECKS:	
ACTION REQUIRED:	
INSPECTION TIME:	INSPECTED BY:
COMMENTS:	

DATE:	SERIAL NUMBER:
LOCATION:	
ALARM CHECKS:	
ACTION REQUIRED:	
INSPECTION TIME:	INSPECTED BY:
COMMENTS:	

DATE:	SERIAL NUMBER:
LOCATION:	
ALARM CHECKS:	
ACTION REQUIRED:	
INSPECTION TIME:	INSPECTED BY:
COMMENTS:	

DATE:	SERIAL NUMBER:
LOCATION:	
ALARM CHECKS:	
ACTION REQUIRED:	
INSPECTION TIME:	INSPECTED BY:
COMMENTS:	

Fire Alarm Log Book

DATE:	SERIAL NUMBER:
LOCATION:	
ALARM CHECKS:	
ACTION REQUIRED:	
INSPECTION TIME:	INSPECTED BY:
COMMENTS:	

DATE:	SERIAL NUMBER:
LOCATION:	
ALARM CHECKS:	
ACTION REQUIRED:	
INSPECTION TIME:	INSPECTED BY:
COMMENTS:	

DATE:	SERIAL NUMBER:
LOCATION:	
ALARM CHECKS:	
ACTION REQUIRED:	
INSPECTION TIME:	INSPECTED BY:
COMMENTS:	

DATE:	SERIAL NUMBER:
LOCATION:	
ALARM CHECKS:	
ACTION REQUIRED:	
INSPECTION TIME:	INSPECTED BY:
COMMENTS:	

Fire Alarm Log Book

DATE:	SERIAL NUMBER:
LOCATION:	
ALARM CHECKS:	
ACTION REQUIRED:	
INSPECTION TIME:	INSPECTED BY:
COMMENTS:	

DATE:	SERIAL NUMBER:
LOCATION:	
ALARM CHECKS:	
ACTION REQUIRED:	
INSPECTION TIME:	INSPECTED BY:
COMMENTS:	

DATE:	SERIAL NUMBER:
LOCATION:	
ALARM CHECKS:	
ACTION REQUIRED:	
INSPECTION TIME:	INSPECTED BY:
COMMENTS:	

DATE:	SERIAL NUMBER:
LOCATION:	
ALARM CHECKS:	
ACTION REQUIRED:	
INSPECTION TIME:	INSPECTED BY:
COMMENTS:	

Fire Alarm Log Book

DATE:	SERIAL NUMBER:
LOCATION:	
ALARM CHECKS:	
ACTION REQUIRED:	
INSPECTION TIME:	INSPECTED BY:
COMMENTS:	

DATE:	SERIAL NUMBER:
LOCATION:	
ALARM CHECKS:	
ACTION REQUIRED:	
INSPECTION TIME:	INSPECTED BY:
COMMENTS:	

DATE:	SERIAL NUMBER:
LOCATION:	
ALARM CHECKS:	
ACTION REQUIRED:	
INSPECTION TIME:	INSPECTED BY:
COMMENTS:	

DATE:	SERIAL NUMBER:
LOCATION:	
ALARM CHECKS:	
ACTION REQUIRED:	
INSPECTION TIME:	INSPECTED BY:
COMMENTS:	

Fire Alarm Log Book

DATE:	SERIAL NUMBER:
LOCATION:	
ALARM CHECKS:	
ACTION REQUIRED:	
INSPECTION TIME:	INSPECTED BY:
COMMENTS:	

DATE:	SERIAL NUMBER:
LOCATION:	
ALARM CHECKS:	
ACTION REQUIRED:	
INSPECTION TIME:	INSPECTED BY:
COMMENTS:	

DATE:	SERIAL NUMBER:
LOCATION:	
ALARM CHECKS:	
ACTION REQUIRED:	
INSPECTION TIME:	INSPECTED BY:
COMMENTS:	

DATE:	SERIAL NUMBER:
LOCATION:	
ALARM CHECKS:	
ACTION REQUIRED:	
INSPECTION TIME:	INSPECTED BY:
COMMENTS:	

Fire Alarm Log Book

DATE:	SERIAL NUMBER:
LOCATION:	
ALARM CHECKS:	
ACTION REQUIRED:	
INSPECTION TIME:	INSPECTED BY:
COMMENTS:	

DATE:	SERIAL NUMBER:
LOCATION:	
ALARM CHECKS:	
ACTION REQUIRED:	
INSPECTION TIME:	INSPECTED BY:
COMMENTS:	

DATE:	SERIAL NUMBER:
LOCATION:	
ALARM CHECKS:	
ACTION REQUIRED:	
INSPECTION TIME:	INSPECTED BY:
COMMENTS:	

DATE:	SERIAL NUMBER:
LOCATION:	
ALARM CHECKS:	
ACTION REQUIRED:	
INSPECTION TIME:	INSPECTED BY:
COMMENTS:	

Fire Alarm Log Book

DATE:	SERIAL NUMBER:
LOCATION:	
ALARM CHECKS:	
ACTION REQUIRED:	
INSPECTION TIME:	INSPECTED BY:
COMMENTS:	

DATE:	SERIAL NUMBER:
LOCATION:	
ALARM CHECKS:	
ACTION REQUIRED:	
INSPECTION TIME:	INSPECTED BY:
COMMENTS:	

DATE:	SERIAL NUMBER:
LOCATION:	
ALARM CHECKS:	
ACTION REQUIRED:	
INSPECTION TIME:	INSPECTED BY:
COMMENTS:	

DATE:	SERIAL NUMBER:
LOCATION:	
ALARM CHECKS:	
ACTION REQUIRED:	
INSPECTION TIME:	INSPECTED BY:
COMMENTS:	

Fire Alarm Log Book

DATE:	SERIAL NUMBER:
LOCATION:	
ALARM CHECKS:	
ACTION REQUIRED:	
INSPECTION TIME:	INSPECTED BY:
COMMENTS:	

DATE:	SERIAL NUMBER:
LOCATION:	
ALARM CHECKS:	
ACTION REQUIRED:	
INSPECTION TIME:	INSPECTED BY:
COMMENTS:	

DATE:	SERIAL NUMBER:
LOCATION:	
ALARM CHECKS:	
ACTION REQUIRED:	
INSPECTION TIME:	INSPECTED BY:
COMMENTS:	

DATE:	SERIAL NUMBER:
LOCATION:	
ALARM CHECKS:	
ACTION REQUIRED:	
INSPECTION TIME:	INSPECTED BY:
COMMENTS:	

Fire Alarm Log Book

DATE:	SERIAL NUMBER:
LOCATION:	
ALARM CHECKS:	
ACTION REQUIRED:	
INSPECTION TIME:	INSPECTED BY:
COMMENTS:	

DATE:	SERIAL NUMBER:
LOCATION:	
ALARM CHECKS:	
ACTION REQUIRED:	
INSPECTION TIME:	INSPECTED BY:
COMMENTS:	

DATE:	SERIAL NUMBER:
LOCATION:	
ALARM CHECKS:	
ACTION REQUIRED:	
INSPECTION TIME:	INSPECTED BY:
COMMENTS:	

DATE:	SERIAL NUMBER:
LOCATION:	
ALARM CHECKS:	
ACTION REQUIRED:	
INSPECTION TIME:	INSPECTED BY:
COMMENTS:	

Fire Alarm Log Book

DATE:	SERIAL NUMBER:
LOCATION:	
ALARM CHECKS:	
ACTION REQUIRED:	
INSPECTION TIME:	INSPECTED BY:
COMMENTS:	

DATE:	SERIAL NUMBER:
LOCATION:	
ALARM CHECKS:	
ACTION REQUIRED:	
INSPECTION TIME:	INSPECTED BY:
COMMENTS:	

DATE:	SERIAL NUMBER:
LOCATION:	
ALARM CHECKS:	
ACTION REQUIRED:	
INSPECTION TIME:	INSPECTED BY:
COMMENTS:	

DATE:	SERIAL NUMBER:
LOCATION:	
ALARM CHECKS:	
ACTION REQUIRED:	
INSPECTION TIME:	INSPECTED BY:
COMMENTS:	

Fire Alarm Log Book

DATE:	SERIAL NUMBER:
LOCATION:	
ALARM CHECKS:	
ACTION REQUIRED:	
INSPECTION TIME:	INSPECTED BY:
COMMENTS:	

DATE:	SERIAL NUMBER:
LOCATION:	
ALARM CHECKS:	
ACTION REQUIRED:	
INSPECTION TIME:	INSPECTED BY:
COMMENTS:	

DATE:	SERIAL NUMBER:
LOCATION:	
ALARM CHECKS:	
ACTION REQUIRED:	
INSPECTION TIME:	INSPECTED BY:
COMMENTS:	

DATE:	SERIAL NUMBER:
LOCATION:	
ALARM CHECKS:	
ACTION REQUIRED:	
INSPECTION TIME:	INSPECTED BY:
COMMENTS:	

Fire Alarm Log Book

DATE:	SERIAL NUMBER:
LOCATION:	
ALARM CHECKS:	
ACTION REQUIRED:	
INSPECTION TIME:	INSPECTED BY:
COMMENTS:	

DATE:	SERIAL NUMBER:
LOCATION:	
ALARM CHECKS:	
ACTION REQUIRED:	
INSPECTION TIME:	INSPECTED BY:
COMMENTS:	

DATE:	SERIAL NUMBER:
LOCATION:	
ALARM CHECKS:	
ACTION REQUIRED:	
INSPECTION TIME:	INSPECTED BY:
COMMENTS:	

DATE:	SERIAL NUMBER:
LOCATION:	
ALARM CHECKS:	
ACTION REQUIRED:	
INSPECTION TIME:	INSPECTED BY:
COMMENTS:	

Fire Alarm Log Book

DATE:	SERIAL NUMBER:
LOCATION:	
ALARM CHECKS:	
ACTION REQUIRED:	
INSPECTION TIME:	INSPECTED BY:
COMMENTS:	

DATE:	SERIAL NUMBER:
LOCATION:	
ALARM CHECKS:	
ACTION REQUIRED:	
INSPECTION TIME:	INSPECTED BY:
COMMENTS:	

DATE:	SERIAL NUMBER:
LOCATION:	
ALARM CHECKS:	
ACTION REQUIRED:	
INSPECTION TIME:	INSPECTED BY:
COMMENTS:	

DATE:	SERIAL NUMBER:
LOCATION:	
ALARM CHECKS:	
ACTION REQUIRED:	
INSPECTION TIME:	INSPECTED BY:
COMMENTS:	

Fire Alarm Log Book

DATE:	SERIAL NUMBER:
LOCATION:	
ALARM CHECKS:	
ACTION REQUIRED:	
INSPECTION TIME:	INSPECTED BY:
COMMENTS:	

DATE:	SERIAL NUMBER:
LOCATION:	
ALARM CHECKS:	
ACTION REQUIRED:	
INSPECTION TIME:	INSPECTED BY:
COMMENTS:	

DATE:	SERIAL NUMBER:
LOCATION:	
ALARM CHECKS:	
ACTION REQUIRED:	
INSPECTION TIME:	INSPECTED BY:
COMMENTS:	

DATE:	SERIAL NUMBER:
LOCATION:	
ALARM CHECKS:	
ACTION REQUIRED:	
INSPECTION TIME:	INSPECTED BY:
COMMENTS:	

Fire Alarm Log Book

DATE:	SERIAL NUMBER:
LOCATION:	
ALARM CHECKS:	
ACTION REQUIRED:	
INSPECTION TIME:	INSPECTED BY:
COMMENTS:	

DATE:	SERIAL NUMBER:
LOCATION:	
ALARM CHECKS:	
ACTION REQUIRED:	
INSPECTION TIME:	INSPECTED BY:
COMMENTS:	

DATE:	SERIAL NUMBER:
LOCATION:	
ALARM CHECKS:	
ACTION REQUIRED:	
INSPECTION TIME:	INSPECTED BY:
COMMENTS:	

DATE:	SERIAL NUMBER:
LOCATION:	
ALARM CHECKS:	
ACTION REQUIRED:	
INSPECTION TIME:	INSPECTED BY:
COMMENTS:	

Fire Alarm Log Book

DATE:	SERIAL NUMBER:
LOCATION:	
ALARM CHECKS:	
ACTION REQUIRED:	
INSPECTION TIME:	INSPECTED BY:
COMMENTS:	

DATE:	SERIAL NUMBER:
LOCATION:	
ALARM CHECKS:	
ACTION REQUIRED:	
INSPECTION TIME:	INSPECTED BY:
COMMENTS:	

DATE:	SERIAL NUMBER:
LOCATION:	
ALARM CHECKS:	
ACTION REQUIRED:	
INSPECTION TIME:	INSPECTED BY:
COMMENTS:	

DATE:	SERIAL NUMBER:
LOCATION:	
ALARM CHECKS:	
ACTION REQUIRED:	
INSPECTION TIME:	INSPECTED BY:
COMMENTS:	

Fire Alarm Log Book

DATE:	SERIAL NUMBER:
LOCATION:	
ALARM CHECKS:	
ACTION REQUIRED:	
INSPECTION TIME:	INSPECTED BY:
COMMENTS:	

DATE:	SERIAL NUMBER:
LOCATION:	
ALARM CHECKS:	
ACTION REQUIRED:	
INSPECTION TIME:	INSPECTED BY:
COMMENTS:	

DATE:	SERIAL NUMBER:
LOCATION:	
ALARM CHECKS:	
ACTION REQUIRED:	
INSPECTION TIME:	INSPECTED BY:
COMMENTS:	

DATE:	SERIAL NUMBER:
LOCATION:	
ALARM CHECKS:	
ACTION REQUIRED:	
INSPECTION TIME:	INSPECTED BY:
COMMENTS:	

Fire Alarm Log Book

DATE:	SERIAL NUMBER:
LOCATION:	
ALARM CHECKS:	
ACTION REQUIRED:	
INSPECTION TIME:	INSPECTED BY:
COMMENTS:	

DATE:	SERIAL NUMBER:
LOCATION:	
ALARM CHECKS:	
ACTION REQUIRED:	
INSPECTION TIME:	INSPECTED BY:
COMMENTS:	

DATE:	SERIAL NUMBER:
LOCATION:	
ALARM CHECKS:	
ACTION REQUIRED:	
INSPECTION TIME:	INSPECTED BY:
COMMENTS:	

DATE:	SERIAL NUMBER:
LOCATION:	
ALARM CHECKS:	
ACTION REQUIRED:	
INSPECTION TIME:	INSPECTED BY:
COMMENTS:	

Fire Alarm Log Book

DATE:	SERIAL NUMBER:
LOCATION:	
ALARM CHECKS:	
ACTION REQUIRED:	
INSPECTION TIME:	INSPECTED BY:
COMMENTS:	

DATE:	SERIAL NUMBER:
LOCATION:	
ALARM CHECKS:	
ACTION REQUIRED:	
INSPECTION TIME:	INSPECTED BY:
COMMENTS:	

DATE:	SERIAL NUMBER:
LOCATION:	
ALARM CHECKS:	
ACTION REQUIRED:	
INSPECTION TIME:	INSPECTED BY:
COMMENTS:	

DATE:	SERIAL NUMBER:
LOCATION:	
ALARM CHECKS:	
ACTION REQUIRED:	
INSPECTION TIME:	INSPECTED BY:
COMMENTS:	

Fire Alarm Log Book

DATE:	SERIAL NUMBER:
LOCATION:	
ALARM CHECKS:	
ACTION REQUIRED:	
INSPECTION TIME:	INSPECTED BY:
COMMENTS:	

DATE:	SERIAL NUMBER:
LOCATION:	
ALARM CHECKS:	
ACTION REQUIRED:	
INSPECTION TIME:	INSPECTED BY:
COMMENTS:	

DATE:	SERIAL NUMBER:
LOCATION:	
ALARM CHECKS:	
ACTION REQUIRED:	
INSPECTION TIME:	INSPECTED BY:
COMMENTS:	

DATE:	SERIAL NUMBER:
LOCATION:	
ALARM CHECKS:	
ACTION REQUIRED:	
INSPECTION TIME:	INSPECTED BY:
COMMENTS:	

Fire Alarm Log Book

DATE:	SERIAL NUMBER:
LOCATION:	
ALARM CHECKS:	
ACTION REQUIRED:	
INSPECTION TIME:	INSPECTED BY:
COMMENTS:	

DATE:	SERIAL NUMBER:
LOCATION:	
ALARM CHECKS:	
ACTION REQUIRED:	
INSPECTION TIME:	INSPECTED BY:
COMMENTS:	

DATE:	SERIAL NUMBER:
LOCATION:	
ALARM CHECKS:	
ACTION REQUIRED:	
INSPECTION TIME:	INSPECTED BY:
COMMENTS:	

DATE:	SERIAL NUMBER:
LOCATION:	
ALARM CHECKS:	
ACTION REQUIRED:	
INSPECTION TIME:	INSPECTED BY:
COMMENTS:	

Fire Alarm Log Book

DATE:	SERIAL NUMBER:
LOCATION:	
ALARM CHECKS:	
ACTION REQUIRED:	
INSPECTION TIME:	INSPECTED BY:
COMMENTS:	

DATE:	SERIAL NUMBER:
LOCATION:	
ALARM CHECKS:	
ACTION REQUIRED:	
INSPECTION TIME:	INSPECTED BY:
COMMENTS:	

DATE:	SERIAL NUMBER:
LOCATION:	
ALARM CHECKS:	
ACTION REQUIRED:	
INSPECTION TIME:	INSPECTED BY:
COMMENTS:	

DATE:	SERIAL NUMBER:
LOCATION:	
ALARM CHECKS:	
ACTION REQUIRED:	
INSPECTION TIME:	INSPECTED BY:
COMMENTS:	

Fire Alarm Log Book

DATE:	SERIAL NUMBER:
LOCATION:	
ALARM CHECKS:	
ACTION REQUIRED:	
INSPECTION TIME:	INSPECTED BY:
COMMENTS:	

DATE:	SERIAL NUMBER:
LOCATION:	
ALARM CHECKS:	
ACTION REQUIRED:	
INSPECTION TIME:	INSPECTED BY:
COMMENTS:	

DATE:	SERIAL NUMBER:
LOCATION:	
ALARM CHECKS:	
ACTION REQUIRED:	
INSPECTION TIME:	INSPECTED BY:
COMMENTS:	

DATE:	SERIAL NUMBER:
LOCATION:	
ALARM CHECKS:	
ACTION REQUIRED:	
INSPECTION TIME:	INSPECTED BY:
COMMENTS:	

Fire Alarm Log Book

DATE:	SERIAL NUMBER:
LOCATION:	
ALARM CHECKS:	
ACTION REQUIRED:	
INSPECTION TIME:	INSPECTED BY:
COMMENTS:	

DATE:	SERIAL NUMBER:
LOCATION:	
ALARM CHECKS:	
ACTION REQUIRED:	
INSPECTION TIME:	INSPECTED BY:
COMMENTS:	

DATE:	SERIAL NUMBER:
LOCATION:	
ALARM CHECKS:	
ACTION REQUIRED:	
INSPECTION TIME:	INSPECTED BY:
COMMENTS:	

DATE:	SERIAL NUMBER:
LOCATION:	
ALARM CHECKS:	
ACTION REQUIRED:	
INSPECTION TIME:	INSPECTED BY:
COMMENTS:	

Fire Alarm Log Book

DATE:	SERIAL NUMBER:
LOCATION:	
ALARM CHECKS:	
ACTION REQUIRED:	
INSPECTION TIME:	INSPECTED BY:
COMMENTS:	

DATE:	SERIAL NUMBER:
LOCATION:	
ALARM CHECKS:	
ACTION REQUIRED:	
INSPECTION TIME:	INSPECTED BY:
COMMENTS:	

DATE:	SERIAL NUMBER:
LOCATION:	
ALARM CHECKS:	
ACTION REQUIRED:	
INSPECTION TIME:	INSPECTED BY:
COMMENTS:	

DATE:	SERIAL NUMBER:
LOCATION:	
ALARM CHECKS:	
ACTION REQUIRED:	
INSPECTION TIME:	INSPECTED BY:
COMMENTS:	

Fire Alarm Log Book

DATE:	SERIAL NUMBER:
LOCATION:	
ALARM CHECKS:	
ACTION REQUIRED:	
INSPECTION TIME:	INSPECTED BY:
COMMENTS:	

DATE:	SERIAL NUMBER:
LOCATION:	
ALARM CHECKS:	
ACTION REQUIRED:	
INSPECTION TIME:	INSPECTED BY:
COMMENTS:	

DATE:	SERIAL NUMBER:
LOCATION:	
ALARM CHECKS:	
ACTION REQUIRED:	
INSPECTION TIME:	INSPECTED BY:
COMMENTS:	

DATE:	SERIAL NUMBER:
LOCATION:	
ALARM CHECKS:	
ACTION REQUIRED:	
INSPECTION TIME:	INSPECTED BY:
COMMENTS:	

Fire Alarm Log Book

DATE:	SERIAL NUMBER:
LOCATION:	
ALARM CHECKS:	
ACTION REQUIRED:	
INSPECTION TIME:	INSPECTED BY:
COMMENTS:	

DATE:	SERIAL NUMBER:
LOCATION:	
ALARM CHECKS:	
ACTION REQUIRED:	
INSPECTION TIME:	INSPECTED BY:
COMMENTS:	

DATE:	SERIAL NUMBER:
LOCATION:	
ALARM CHECKS:	
ACTION REQUIRED:	
INSPECTION TIME:	INSPECTED BY:
COMMENTS:	

DATE:	SERIAL NUMBER:
LOCATION:	
ALARM CHECKS:	
ACTION REQUIRED:	
INSPECTION TIME:	INSPECTED BY:
COMMENTS:	

Fire Alarm Log Book

DATE:	SERIAL NUMBER:
LOCATION:	
ALARM CHECKS:	
ACTION REQUIRED:	
INSPECTION TIME:	INSPECTED BY:
COMMENTS:	

DATE:	SERIAL NUMBER:
LOCATION:	
ALARM CHECKS:	
ACTION REQUIRED:	
INSPECTION TIME:	INSPECTED BY:
COMMENTS:	

DATE:	SERIAL NUMBER:
LOCATION:	
ALARM CHECKS:	
ACTION REQUIRED:	
INSPECTION TIME:	INSPECTED BY:
COMMENTS:	

DATE:	SERIAL NUMBER:
LOCATION:	
ALARM CHECKS:	
ACTION REQUIRED:	
INSPECTION TIME:	INSPECTED BY:
COMMENTS:	

Fire Alarm Log Book

DATE:	SERIAL NUMBER:
LOCATION:	
ALARM CHECKS:	
ACTION REQUIRED:	
INSPECTION TIME:	INSPECTED BY:
COMMENTS:	

DATE:	SERIAL NUMBER:
LOCATION:	
ALARM CHECKS:	
ACTION REQUIRED:	
INSPECTION TIME:	INSPECTED BY:
COMMENTS:	

DATE:	SERIAL NUMBER:
LOCATION:	
ALARM CHECKS:	
ACTION REQUIRED:	
INSPECTION TIME:	INSPECTED BY:
COMMENTS:	

DATE:	SERIAL NUMBER:
LOCATION:	
ALARM CHECKS:	
ACTION REQUIRED:	
INSPECTION TIME:	INSPECTED BY:
COMMENTS:	

Fire Alarm Log Book

DATE:	SERIAL NUMBER:
LOCATION:	
ALARM CHECKS:	
ACTION REQUIRED:	
INSPECTION TIME:	INSPECTED BY:
COMMENTS:	

DATE:	SERIAL NUMBER:
LOCATION:	
ALARM CHECKS:	
ACTION REQUIRED:	
INSPECTION TIME:	INSPECTED BY:
COMMENTS:	

DATE:	SERIAL NUMBER:
LOCATION:	
ALARM CHECKS:	
ACTION REQUIRED:	
INSPECTION TIME:	INSPECTED BY:
COMMENTS:	

DATE:	SERIAL NUMBER:
LOCATION:	
ALARM CHECKS:	
ACTION REQUIRED:	
INSPECTION TIME:	INSPECTED BY:
COMMENTS:	

Fire Alarm Log Book

DATE:	SERIAL NUMBER:
LOCATION:	
ALARM CHECKS:	
ACTION REQUIRED:	
INSPECTION TIME:	INSPECTED BY:
COMMENTS:	

DATE:	SERIAL NUMBER:
LOCATION:	
ALARM CHECKS:	
ACTION REQUIRED:	
INSPECTION TIME:	INSPECTED BY:
COMMENTS:	

DATE:	SERIAL NUMBER:
LOCATION:	
ALARM CHECKS:	
ACTION REQUIRED:	
INSPECTION TIME:	INSPECTED BY:
COMMENTS:	

DATE:	SERIAL NUMBER:
LOCATION:	
ALARM CHECKS:	
ACTION REQUIRED:	
INSPECTION TIME:	INSPECTED BY:
COMMENTS:	

Fire Alarm Log Book

DATE:	SERIAL NUMBER:
LOCATION:	
ALARM CHECKS:	
ACTION REQUIRED:	
INSPECTION TIME:	INSPECTED BY:
COMMENTS:	

DATE:	SERIAL NUMBER:
LOCATION:	
ALARM CHECKS:	
ACTION REQUIRED:	
INSPECTION TIME:	INSPECTED BY:
COMMENTS:	

DATE:	SERIAL NUMBER:
LOCATION:	
ALARM CHECKS:	
ACTION REQUIRED:	
INSPECTION TIME:	INSPECTED BY:
COMMENTS:	

DATE:	SERIAL NUMBER:
LOCATION:	
ALARM CHECKS:	
ACTION REQUIRED:	
INSPECTION TIME:	INSPECTED BY:
COMMENTS:	

Fire Alarm Log Book

DATE:	SERIAL NUMBER:
LOCATION:	
ALARM CHECKS:	
ACTION REQUIRED:	
INSPECTION TIME:	INSPECTED BY:
COMMENTS:	

DATE:	SERIAL NUMBER:
LOCATION:	
ALARM CHECKS:	
ACTION REQUIRED:	
INSPECTION TIME:	INSPECTED BY:
COMMENTS:	

DATE:	SERIAL NUMBER:
LOCATION:	
ALARM CHECKS:	
ACTION REQUIRED:	
INSPECTION TIME:	INSPECTED BY:
COMMENTS:	

DATE:	SERIAL NUMBER:
LOCATION:	
ALARM CHECKS:	
ACTION REQUIRED:	
INSPECTION TIME:	INSPECTED BY:
COMMENTS:	

Fire Alarm Log Book

DATE:	SERIAL NUMBER:
LOCATION:	
ALARM CHECKS:	
ACTION REQUIRED:	
INSPECTION TIME:	INSPECTED BY:
COMMENTS:	

DATE:	SERIAL NUMBER:
LOCATION:	
ALARM CHECKS:	
ACTION REQUIRED:	
INSPECTION TIME:	INSPECTED BY:
COMMENTS:	

DATE:	SERIAL NUMBER:
LOCATION:	
ALARM CHECKS:	
ACTION REQUIRED:	
INSPECTION TIME:	INSPECTED BY:
COMMENTS:	

DATE:	SERIAL NUMBER:
LOCATION:	
ALARM CHECKS:	
ACTION REQUIRED:	
INSPECTION TIME:	INSPECTED BY:
COMMENTS:	

Fire Alarm Log Book

DATE:	SERIAL NUMBER:
LOCATION:	
ALARM CHECKS:	
ACTION REQUIRED:	
INSPECTION TIME:	INSPECTED BY:
COMMENTS:	

DATE:	SERIAL NUMBER:
LOCATION:	
ALARM CHECKS:	
ACTION REQUIRED:	
INSPECTION TIME:	INSPECTED BY:
COMMENTS:	

DATE:	SERIAL NUMBER:
LOCATION:	
ALARM CHECKS:	
ACTION REQUIRED:	
INSPECTION TIME:	INSPECTED BY:
COMMENTS:	

DATE:	SERIAL NUMBER:
LOCATION:	
ALARM CHECKS:	
ACTION REQUIRED:	
INSPECTION TIME:	INSPECTED BY:
COMMENTS:	

Fire Alarm Log Book

DATE:	SERIAL NUMBER:
LOCATION:	
ALARM CHECKS:	
ACTION REQUIRED:	
INSPECTION TIME:	INSPECTED BY:
COMMENTS:	

DATE:	SERIAL NUMBER:
LOCATION:	
ALARM CHECKS:	
ACTION REQUIRED:	
INSPECTION TIME:	INSPECTED BY:
COMMENTS:	

DATE:	SERIAL NUMBER:
LOCATION:	
ALARM CHECKS:	
ACTION REQUIRED:	
INSPECTION TIME:	INSPECTED BY:
COMMENTS:	

DATE:	SERIAL NUMBER:
LOCATION:	
ALARM CHECKS:	
ACTION REQUIRED:	
INSPECTION TIME:	INSPECTED BY:
COMMENTS:	

Fire Alarm Log Book

DATE:	SERIAL NUMBER:
LOCATION:	
ALARM CHECKS:	
ACTION REQUIRED:	
INSPECTION TIME:	INSPECTED BY:
COMMENTS:	

DATE:	SERIAL NUMBER:
LOCATION:	
ALARM CHECKS:	
ACTION REQUIRED:	
INSPECTION TIME:	INSPECTED BY:
COMMENTS:	

DATE:	SERIAL NUMBER:
LOCATION:	
ALARM CHECKS:	
ACTION REQUIRED:	
INSPECTION TIME:	INSPECTED BY:
COMMENTS:	

DATE:	SERIAL NUMBER:
LOCATION:	
ALARM CHECKS:	
ACTION REQUIRED:	
INSPECTION TIME:	INSPECTED BY:
COMMENTS:	

Fire Alarm Log Book

DATE:	SERIAL NUMBER:
LOCATION:	
ALARM CHECKS:	
ACTION REQUIRED:	
INSPECTION TIME:	INSPECTED BY:
COMMENTS:	

DATE:	SERIAL NUMBER:
LOCATION:	
ALARM CHECKS:	
ACTION REQUIRED:	
INSPECTION TIME:	INSPECTED BY:
COMMENTS:	

DATE:	SERIAL NUMBER:
LOCATION:	
ALARM CHECKS:	
ACTION REQUIRED:	
INSPECTION TIME:	INSPECTED BY:
COMMENTS:	

DATE:	SERIAL NUMBER:
LOCATION:	
ALARM CHECKS:	
ACTION REQUIRED:	
INSPECTION TIME:	INSPECTED BY:
COMMENTS:	

Fire Alarm Log Book

DATE:	SERIAL NUMBER:
LOCATION:	
ALARM CHECKS:	
ACTION REQUIRED:	
INSPECTION TIME:	INSPECTED BY:
COMMENTS:	

DATE:	SERIAL NUMBER:
LOCATION:	
ALARM CHECKS:	
ACTION REQUIRED:	
INSPECTION TIME:	INSPECTED BY:
COMMENTS:	

DATE:	SERIAL NUMBER:
LOCATION:	
ALARM CHECKS:	
ACTION REQUIRED:	
INSPECTION TIME:	INSPECTED BY:
COMMENTS:	

DATE:	SERIAL NUMBER:
LOCATION:	
ALARM CHECKS:	
ACTION REQUIRED:	
INSPECTION TIME:	INSPECTED BY:
COMMENTS:	

Fire Alarm Log Book

DATE:	SERIAL NUMBER:
LOCATION:	
ALARM CHECKS:	
ACTION REQUIRED:	
INSPECTION TIME:	INSPECTED BY:
COMMENTS:	

DATE:	SERIAL NUMBER:
LOCATION:	
ALARM CHECKS:	
ACTION REQUIRED:	
INSPECTION TIME:	INSPECTED BY:
COMMENTS:	

DATE:	SERIAL NUMBER:
LOCATION:	
ALARM CHECKS:	
ACTION REQUIRED:	
INSPECTION TIME:	INSPECTED BY:
COMMENTS:	

DATE:	SERIAL NUMBER:
LOCATION:	
ALARM CHECKS:	
ACTION REQUIRED:	
INSPECTION TIME:	INSPECTED BY:
COMMENTS:	

Fire Alarm Log Book

DATE:	SERIAL NUMBER:
LOCATION:	
ALARM CHECKS:	
ACTION REQUIRED:	
INSPECTION TIME:	INSPECTED BY:
COMMENTS:	

DATE:	SERIAL NUMBER:
LOCATION:	
ALARM CHECKS:	
ACTION REQUIRED:	
INSPECTION TIME:	INSPECTED BY:
COMMENTS:	

DATE:	SERIAL NUMBER:
LOCATION:	
ALARM CHECKS:	
ACTION REQUIRED:	
INSPECTION TIME:	INSPECTED BY:
COMMENTS:	

DATE:	SERIAL NUMBER:
LOCATION:	
ALARM CHECKS:	
ACTION REQUIRED:	
INSPECTION TIME:	INSPECTED BY:
COMMENTS:	

Fire Alarm Log Book

DATE:	SERIAL NUMBER:
LOCATION:	
ALARM CHECKS:	
ACTION REQUIRED:	
INSPECTION TIME:	INSPECTED BY:
COMMENTS:	

DATE:	SERIAL NUMBER:
LOCATION:	
ALARM CHECKS:	
ACTION REQUIRED:	
INSPECTION TIME:	INSPECTED BY:
COMMENTS:	

DATE:	SERIAL NUMBER:
LOCATION:	
ALARM CHECKS:	
ACTION REQUIRED:	
INSPECTION TIME:	INSPECTED BY:
COMMENTS:	

DATE:	SERIAL NUMBER:
LOCATION:	
ALARM CHECKS:	
ACTION REQUIRED:	
INSPECTION TIME:	INSPECTED BY:
COMMENTS:	

Fire Alarm Log Book

DATE:	SERIAL NUMBER:
LOCATION:	
ALARM CHECKS:	
ACTION REQUIRED:	
INSPECTION TIME:	INSPECTED BY:
COMMENTS:	

DATE:	SERIAL NUMBER:
LOCATION:	
ALARM CHECKS:	
ACTION REQUIRED:	
INSPECTION TIME:	INSPECTED BY:
COMMENTS:	

DATE:	SERIAL NUMBER:
LOCATION:	
ALARM CHECKS:	
ACTION REQUIRED:	
INSPECTION TIME:	INSPECTED BY:
COMMENTS:	

DATE:	SERIAL NUMBER:
LOCATION:	
ALARM CHECKS:	
ACTION REQUIRED:	
INSPECTION TIME:	INSPECTED BY:
COMMENTS:	

Fire Alarm Log Book

DATE:	SERIAL NUMBER:
LOCATION:	
ALARM CHECKS:	
ACTION REQUIRED:	
INSPECTION TIME:	INSPECTED BY:
COMMENTS:	

DATE:	SERIAL NUMBER:
LOCATION:	
ALARM CHECKS:	
ACTION REQUIRED:	
INSPECTION TIME:	INSPECTED BY:
COMMENTS:	

DATE:	SERIAL NUMBER:
LOCATION:	
ALARM CHECKS:	
ACTION REQUIRED:	
INSPECTION TIME:	INSPECTED BY:
COMMENTS:	

DATE:	SERIAL NUMBER:
LOCATION:	
ALARM CHECKS:	
ACTION REQUIRED:	
INSPECTION TIME:	INSPECTED BY:
COMMENTS:	

Fire Alarm Log Book

DATE:	SERIAL NUMBER:
LOCATION:	
ALARM CHECKS:	
ACTION REQUIRED:	
INSPECTION TIME:	INSPECTED BY:
COMMENTS:	

DATE:	SERIAL NUMBER:
LOCATION:	
ALARM CHECKS:	
ACTION REQUIRED:	
INSPECTION TIME:	INSPECTED BY:
COMMENTS:	

DATE:	SERIAL NUMBER:
LOCATION:	
ALARM CHECKS:	
ACTION REQUIRED:	
INSPECTION TIME:	INSPECTED BY:
COMMENTS:	

DATE:	SERIAL NUMBER:
LOCATION:	
ALARM CHECKS:	
ACTION REQUIRED:	
INSPECTION TIME:	INSPECTED BY:
COMMENTS:	

Fire Alarm Log Book

DATE:	SERIAL NUMBER:
LOCATION:	
ALARM CHECKS:	
ACTION REQUIRED:	
INSPECTION TIME:	INSPECTED BY:
COMMENTS:	

DATE:	SERIAL NUMBER:
LOCATION:	
ALARM CHECKS:	
ACTION REQUIRED:	
INSPECTION TIME:	INSPECTED BY:
COMMENTS:	

DATE:	SERIAL NUMBER:
LOCATION:	
ALARM CHECKS:	
ACTION REQUIRED:	
INSPECTION TIME:	INSPECTED BY:
COMMENTS:	

DATE:	SERIAL NUMBER:
LOCATION:	
ALARM CHECKS:	
ACTION REQUIRED:	
INSPECTION TIME:	INSPECTED BY:
COMMENTS:	

Fire Alarm Log Book

DATE:	SERIAL NUMBER:
LOCATION:	
ALARM CHECKS:	
ACTION REQUIRED:	
INSPECTION TIME:	INSPECTED BY:
COMMENTS:	

DATE:	SERIAL NUMBER:
LOCATION:	
ALARM CHECKS:	
ACTION REQUIRED:	
INSPECTION TIME:	INSPECTED BY:
COMMENTS:	

DATE:	SERIAL NUMBER:
LOCATION:	
ALARM CHECKS:	
ACTION REQUIRED:	
INSPECTION TIME:	INSPECTED BY:
COMMENTS:	

DATE:	SERIAL NUMBER:
LOCATION:	
ALARM CHECKS:	
ACTION REQUIRED:	
INSPECTION TIME:	INSPECTED BY:
COMMENTS:	

Fire Alarm Log Book

DATE:	SERIAL NUMBER:
LOCATION:	
ALARM CHECKS:	
ACTION REQUIRED:	
INSPECTION TIME:	INSPECTED BY:
COMMENTS:	

DATE:	SERIAL NUMBER:
LOCATION:	
ALARM CHECKS:	
ACTION REQUIRED:	
INSPECTION TIME:	INSPECTED BY:
COMMENTS:	

DATE:	SERIAL NUMBER:
LOCATION:	
ALARM CHECKS:	
ACTION REQUIRED:	
INSPECTION TIME:	INSPECTED BY:
COMMENTS:	

DATE:	SERIAL NUMBER:
LOCATION:	
ALARM CHECKS:	
ACTION REQUIRED:	
INSPECTION TIME:	INSPECTED BY:
COMMENTS:	

Fire Alarm Log Book

DATE:	SERIAL NUMBER:
LOCATION:	
ALARM CHECKS:	
ACTION REQUIRED:	
INSPECTION TIME:	INSPECTED BY:
COMMENTS:	

DATE:	SERIAL NUMBER:
LOCATION:	
ALARM CHECKS:	
ACTION REQUIRED:	
INSPECTION TIME:	INSPECTED BY:
COMMENTS:	

DATE:	SERIAL NUMBER:
LOCATION:	
ALARM CHECKS:	
ACTION REQUIRED:	
INSPECTION TIME:	INSPECTED BY:
COMMENTS:	

DATE:	SERIAL NUMBER:
LOCATION:	
ALARM CHECKS:	
ACTION REQUIRED:	
INSPECTION TIME:	INSPECTED BY:
COMMENTS:	

Printed in Great Britain
by Amazon